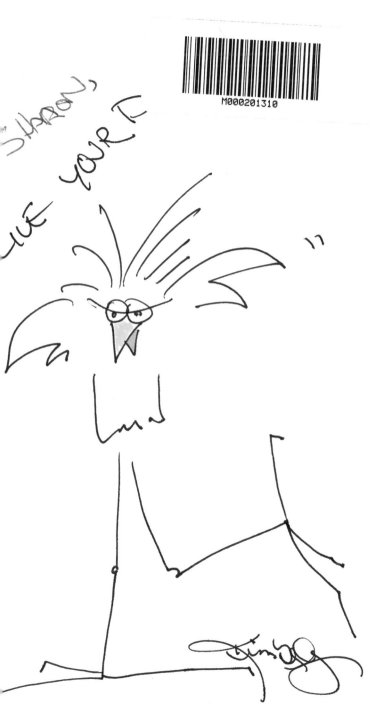

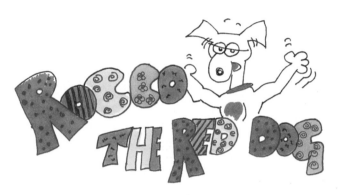

ROCCO THE RED DOG

BY
KIMBERLY MOORE

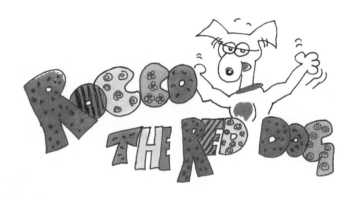

WRITTEN AND ILLUSTRATED
BY
KIMBERLY MOORE

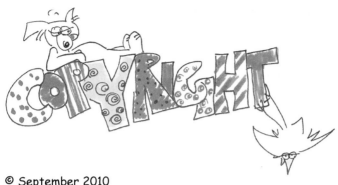

ISBN: 978-0-9829589-4-0
Library of Congress: 2010937603

Published by
INKWELL PRODUCTIONS
Scottsdale, AZ 85254

E-mail: info@inkwellproductions.com
Website: www.inkwellproductions.com

Printed in the United States of America

ROCCO THE RED DOG

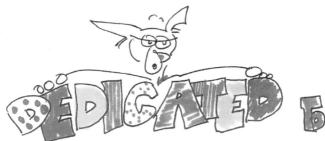

DEDICATED

My Mom Brenda Holben, Whose smile comforts me.

My Dad Robert Moore, Whose strength encourages me.

My 2nd Mom Donna Moore, Who I'm so grateful the Good Lord knew I needed two!

My Sister, Cherylin Hodge, Who always makes me laugh out loud!

My Lil Sister Heather Moore-Kestner, Who is truly blessed! (To be my sister!) :)

My Lil Brother Jay Holben, Who has so much creative talent, and lives his dream! Go Bro!

My Best bff Pamela Jo Cuzick, Whose filled my life with many journeys!

And who makes the Most Delicious Gourmet meals Ever!

My Grandparents who still live in my heart!

My Nephew's, Zachary Hodge, Kyle Hodge, Bobby Hodge, Lincoln Kestner, and Wyatt Kestner.

My Niece, Amberlin Hodge.

Lil Devion Boehnke . . . All, who have grown up with my characters and music. They are all forging their young paths with kind and loving values.

To My next best friends! Kirsten Plambeck, Kathryn Mabry, Carl StJohn and Gina Anglavar. Thank you for lighting my path with joy!

To Nikos Ligidakis my Publisher, Thank you for helping me get my books out of the box and into Life!

I love you all so very much!

ROCCO THE RED DOG

ACKNOWLEDGEMENT

I BELIEVE
WE ARE AFFECTED BY OUR ENVIRONMENT,
THE HOMES WHERE WE GROW, THE PEOPLE
WE MEET AND PLACES WE GO.

I HOPE TO SHARE WARM LIGHT-HEARTED
MESSAGES OF KINDNESS AND HOPE.
WE ALL HAVE GIFTS TO BE SHARED
AND ENCOURAGED.
WE ALL FACE CHALLENGES THAT TEST OUR
TRUE CHARACTER.

WE ALL HAVE AN AMAZING ABILITY TO LEARN & GROW!
BEING AMERICAN, WE CAN DECIDE AT ANY MOMENT
THE KIND OF PERSON WE ARE AND ASPIRE TO BE.
WE CAN DECIDE TO FOSTER OUR NATURAL GIFTS SO
WORK CAN BE MORE LIKE PLAY. IMAGINE THE PRODUCTIVITY
HAPPINESS AND TRUE SUCCESS LIVING TO OUR OWN
POTENTIAL WOULD BE! TEACH SOMEONE TO FIND AND LIVE
IN THEIR TRUTH,
ENCOURAGE THOUGHTFUL CARETAKING OF THEMSELVES
AND TO THOSE ALL AROUND.
WE ARE THE CAPTAINS OF OUR SHIP! WHO AND WHAT
WE ARE, IS A DIRECT RESULT OF WHAT WE THINK.
WHERE OUR HEAD AND HEARTS ARE . . .
OUR FEET WILL FOLLOW.

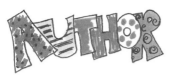

KIMBERLY MOORE WAS BORN IN THE FALL
IN ROCHESTER, NEW YORK.
SHE'S BEEN DRAWING CARTOONS SINCE
SECOND GRADE.
SHE'S PAINTED MURALS IN HOMES, BUSINESSES
AND SCHOOLS.
IN 1986, AT 25 YEARS OLD, KIMBERLY AND
HER BEST BFF PAMELA JO CUZICK OPENED
MASTERPIECE FRAMING. FOR 17 YEARS
THEY THRIVED AND GREW TO BE KNOWN
AS ONE OF THE BEST CRAFTSMAN IN THE
BUSINESS. THEIR WORK IS STILL ENJOYED TODAY.
KIMBERLY MOVED HER HOME AND SHOP TO THE
OUTER NORTH EASTERN EDGE OF SCOTTSDALE,
NEAR NOTHING BUT PEACE AND TRANQUILITY!
"THE RANCH", "THE SPA", "THE COWBOY CORAL",
IS AN EXCELLENT SOURCE OF QUIET CREATIVITY.
THERE, THE NATURE AND SCENERY ARE
REJUVENATING!
THERE, I THINK.
I WRITE.
I AM...

ROCCO THE RED DOG

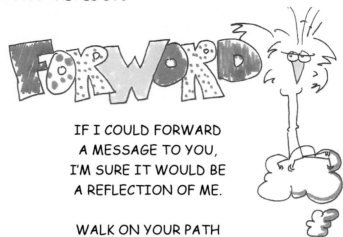

IF I COULD FORWARD
A MESSAGE TO YOU,
I'M SURE IT WOULD BE
A REFLECTION OF ME.

WALK ON YOUR PATH
WITH LOVE IN YOUR HEART.

DISCOVER YOUR DREAMS
IT'S THE BEST PLACE TO START.

CHALLENGES ARE BUMPS
OF OUR FAITH, I'LL SAY

BUT STAY TRUE TO YOUR VALUES
AND LIGHT WILL SHINE YOUR WAY.

ENCOURAGE THE YOUNG, THE OLD
AND THE SMALL.
THERE ARE WONDROUS GIFTS
INSIDE OF US ALL!

I'M ROCCO THE RED DOG
I'M BIG AND STRONG!
I LOVE WAKING UP EARLY
AND GREETING THE DAWN.

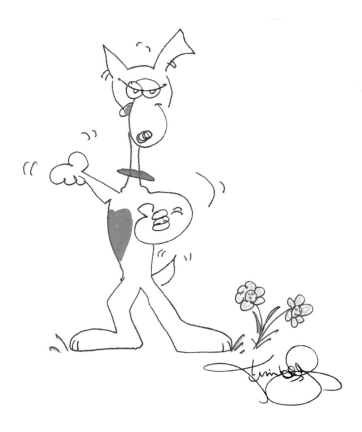

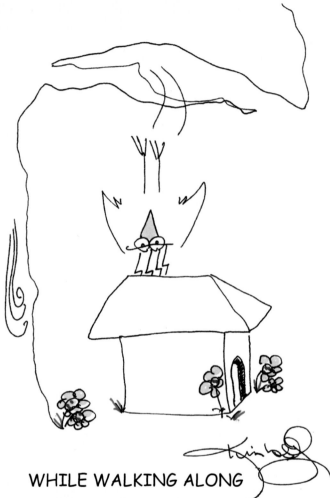

WHILE WALKING ALONG
SINGING MY SONG
PEEP PLOPPED FROM THE SKY
ON MY HOME, UPSIDE DOWN!

WHY DID YOU FLY FROM
THE SKY UPSIDE DOWN?
TWIRLING AND WHIRLING
YOU COULD BREAK YOUR CROWN!

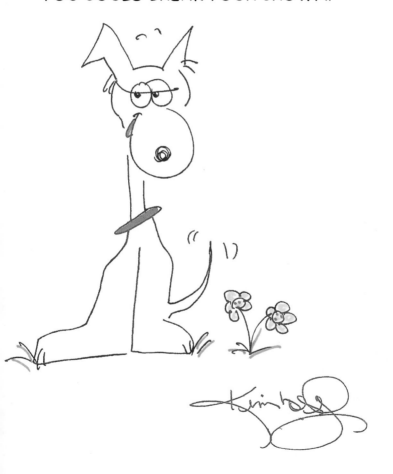

PEEP WAS ASLEEP
WHEN THE WIND BLEW AWAY
THE NEST WHERE HE RESTS
NOW WHERE WOULD HE STAY?

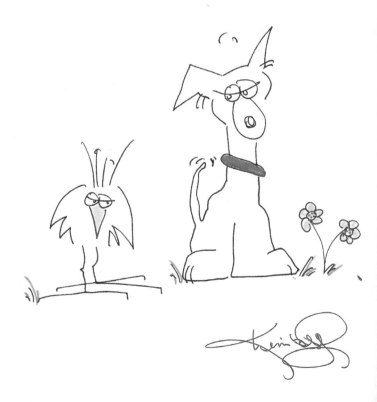

DON'T WORRY PEEP
I'M BIG AND STRONG
YOU'RE MY BEST FRIEND
AND WE GET ALONG!

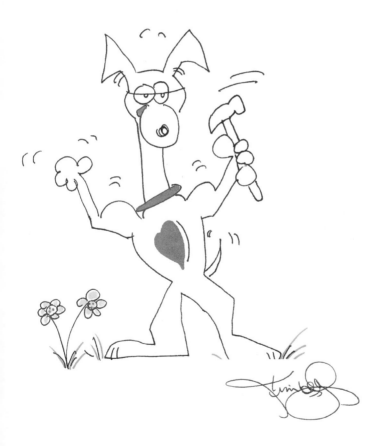

GATHER YOUR FLOCK AND
BIRDS OF A FEATHER,
NOTHING'S TOO HARD
WHILE WORKING TOGETHER!

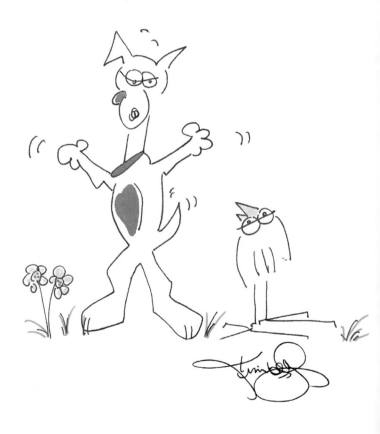

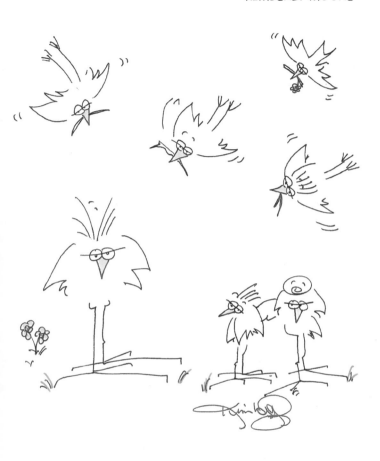

PEEP, PLEASE TELL ROCCO
WE LOST OUR HOMES TOO!
WE'RE REALLY SCARED
AND NOT SURE WHAT TO DO.

COME MY LIL' FRIENDS
WE'LL BUILD ONE AT A TIME
THE BEST NESTS EVER,
ANYONE COULD FIND.

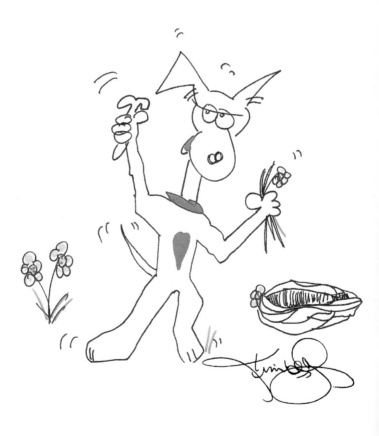

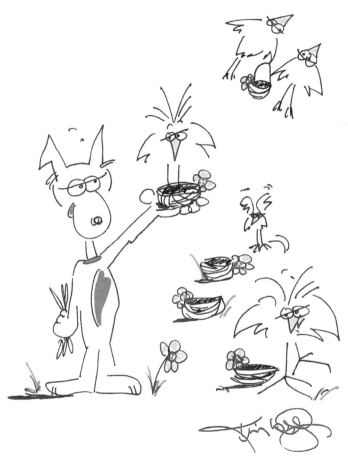

WORKING ALL DAY
WAS MORE LIKE PLAY.
ANY JOB THAT YOU DO
IS WORTH DOING WELL!

SUNSET HAD COME
EVERY BIRD HAD A HOME,
ROCCO SMILED WITH A GLEAM IN HIS EYE
WATCHING HIS BIRD FRIENDS
CHIRP AND FLY!

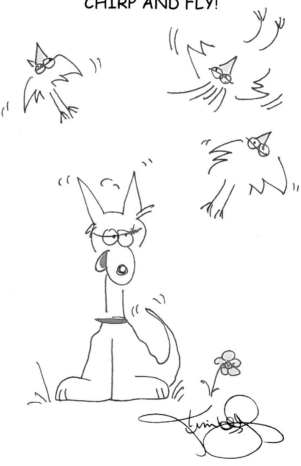

FREE AS A BIRD
ROCCO WISHES HE COULD
FLY THRU THE SKY
ON THE WIND SPREADING GOOD!

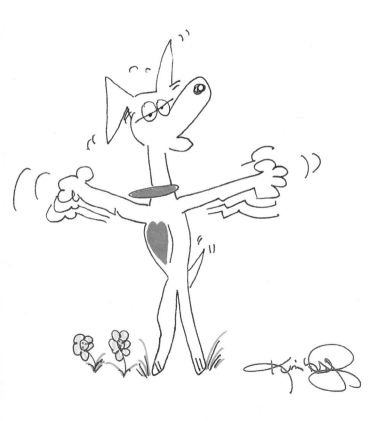

WHEN PEEP SAW ROCCO
AND HEARD OF HIS DREAM,
HE GOT AN IDEA
TO SHOW HIM THE SCENE.

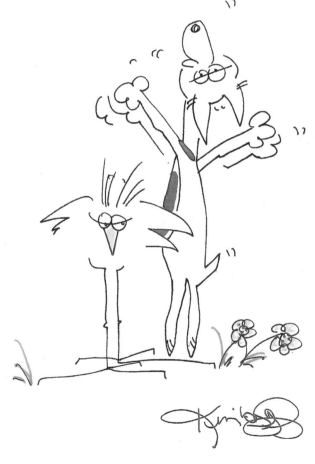

I'M ROCCO THE RED DOG
I'M BIG AND STRONG
KNOWING MY FEET
BELONG ON THE GROUND.

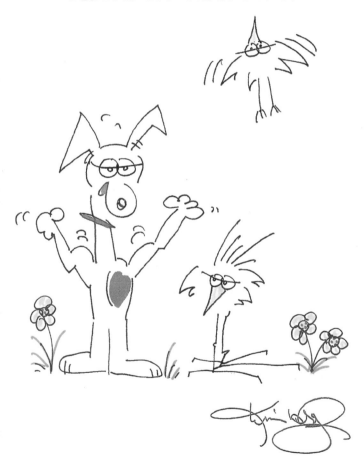

BUT MY HEAD AND MY HEART
ARE FLYING AROUND,
IF I WERE YOU
I'D NEVER COME DOWN.

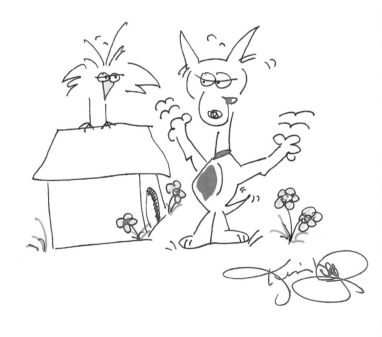

PEEP SPREAD THE WORD
AND IT DIDN'T TAKE LONG
TILL ROCCO'S WISHES
WE'RE ALL OVER TOWN.

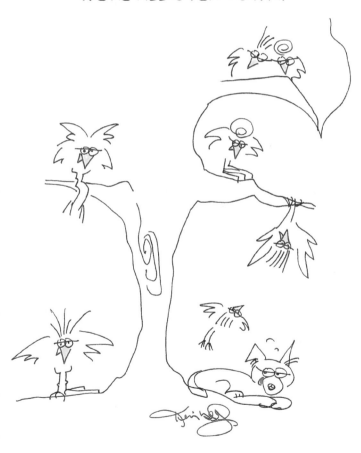

IN FIVE MINUTES FLAT
THREE COUNTIES WIDE
BIRDS WERE ARRIVING
TO GIVE ROCCO A RIDE!

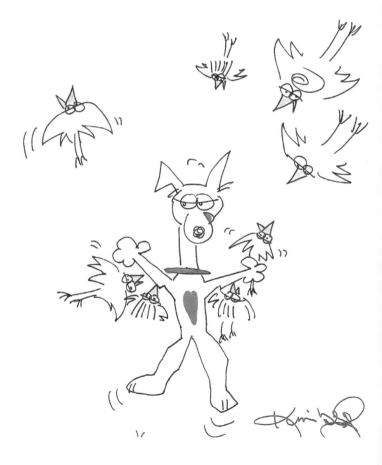

ROCCO WAS PICKED UP
AND CARRIED THROUGH TOWN
UP IN THE CLOUDS
ON THE WIND HE WAS BOUND!

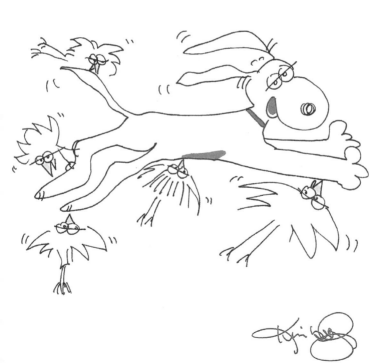

ROCCO WAS TOO HEAVY
FOR A FEW BIRDS TO FLY.
SO BIRD TEAMS WOULD TAKE TURNS
SAILING THE SKY.

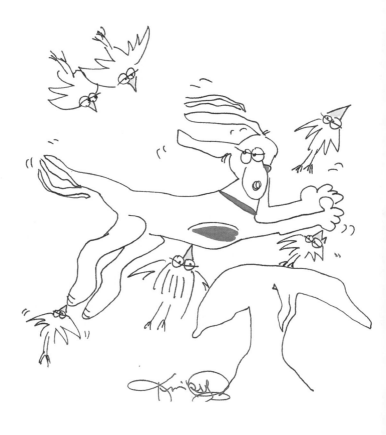

EVERY BIRD THERE
GAVE ROCCO A RIDE.
TAKING THEIR TURN
SMILING INSIDE.

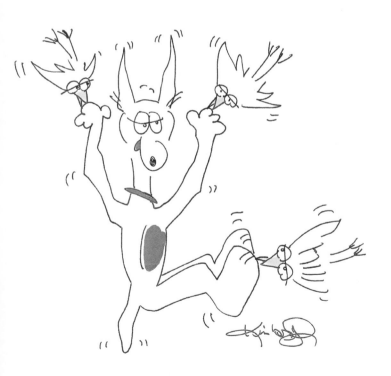

WHEN PEEP AND HIS FRIENDS
SET ROCCO BACK DOWN,
ROCCO WAS SO TICKLED
HE KEPT DANCING ROUND!

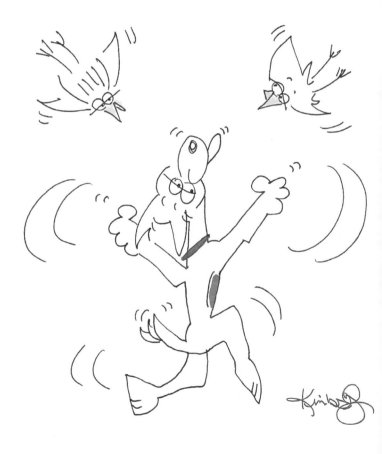

WOW, WHAT A DAY!
WE WORKED AND WE PLAYED
I SAW A NEW WORLD
WITH THE FRIENDS THAT WE MADE.

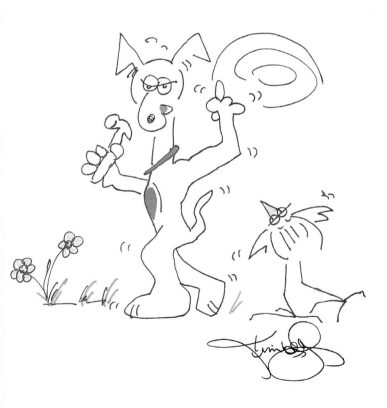

ALTHOUGH YOU'RE NOT TALL,
YOU'RE NOT AT ALL SMALL!
WITH THE STRENGTH THAT YOU HAVE
<u>YOU</u> HAVE IT <u>ALL</u>!

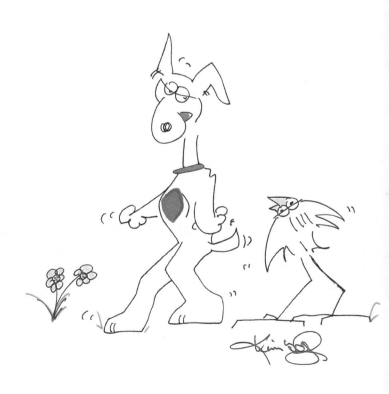

THE GIFTS FROM THE DAY
WILL DANCE IN MY HEAD.
KNOWING TONIGHT YOU'LL
BE SAFE IN YOUR BED.

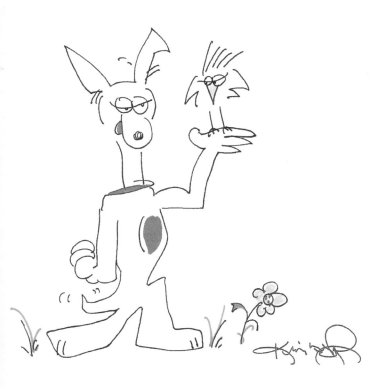

LOVE IS THE PATH THAT I CHOOSE
AND I VALUE.
LIVING IN TRUTH IS THE ROAD
THAT I TRAVEL.

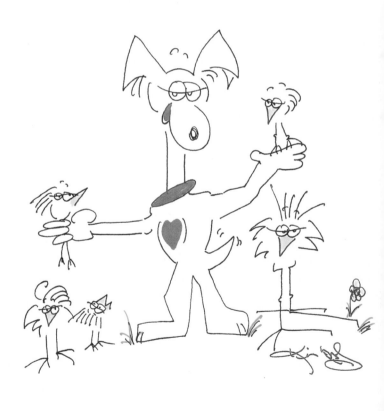

IF ON YOUR JOURNEY
YOU COME TO MY DOOR,
YOU CAN BE YOU
OR IMAGINE MUCH MORE!

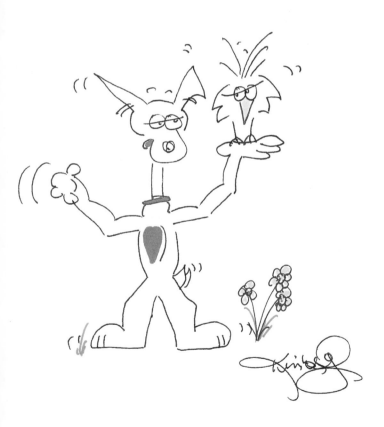

SHARE WHAT YOU LOVE
AND MAKES YOUR HEART SING.
BELIEVE IN YOUR DREAMS
AND DOING YOUR OWN THING.

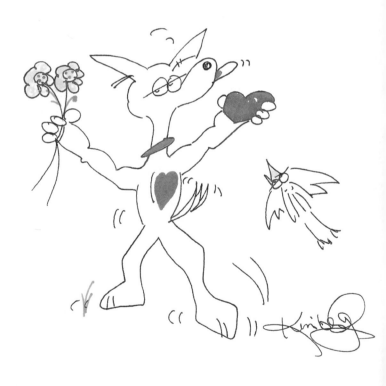

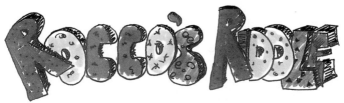

If I Won A Million Dollars,
Without My Friends and Family
To Share It With, I wouldn't
be any Richer or Wiser than I am.
I wouldn't have any more Natural Gifts.
I couldn't grow One Day Younger
or buy One Day Longer.

If I wrote a message on Every Dollar
and Gave it All Away . . .
All you have to do
to receive your Wish Come True
is read it and BELIEVE.
What would your Secret Wish be?
Write it down on a Dollar
and Send It To Me.
If years later, on a Dollar you read
Someone's Wish had come True
you know . . . you BELIEVE
cuz, the WISH IN YOUR HAND,
WAS SENT IN BY YOU!

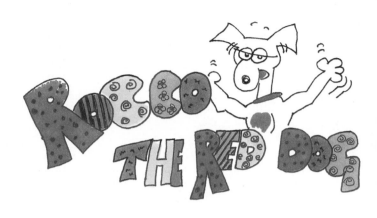

Written and Illustrated
by
Kimberly Moore
7-23-2010

Kimberly Moore
29721 N. 142nd Place
Scottsdale, AZ 85262
480-683-1233

COLLECT:
BOOKS · CD'S · T-SHIRTS · CARDS · HATS · PJ'S · ERASERS
STICKERS · BOOK MARKERS · RUBBER ARM BANDS.